GLUTEN-FREE SLOW COOKER COOKBOOK

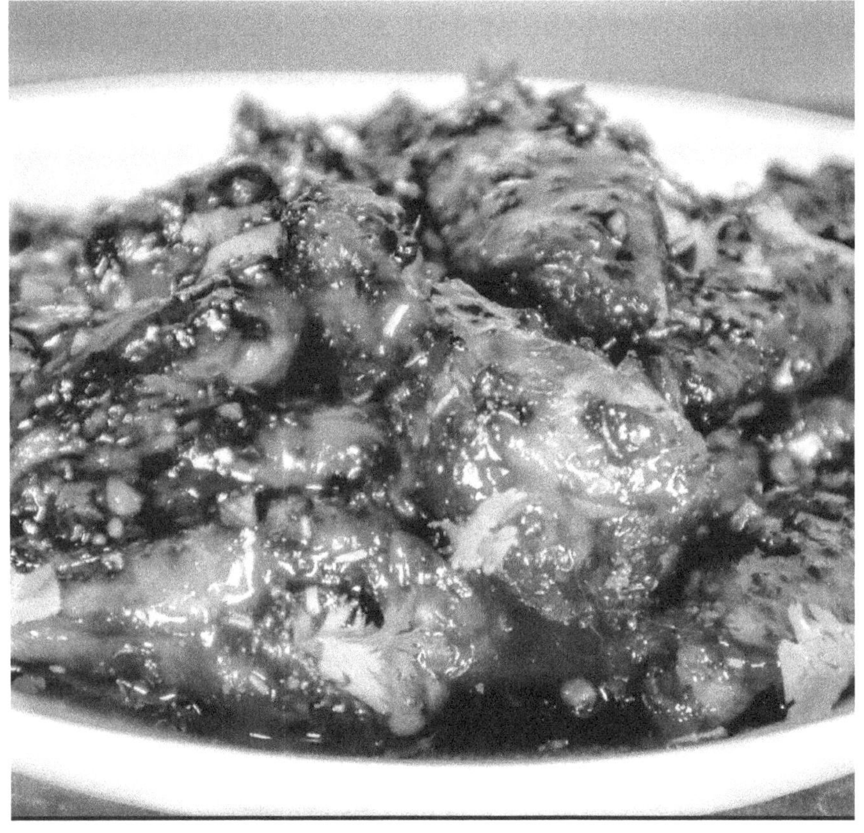

LORENE PEACHEY

TO GAIN ACCESS TO MORE BOOK BY THE AUTHOR SCAN THE QR CODE

TABLE OF CONTENTS

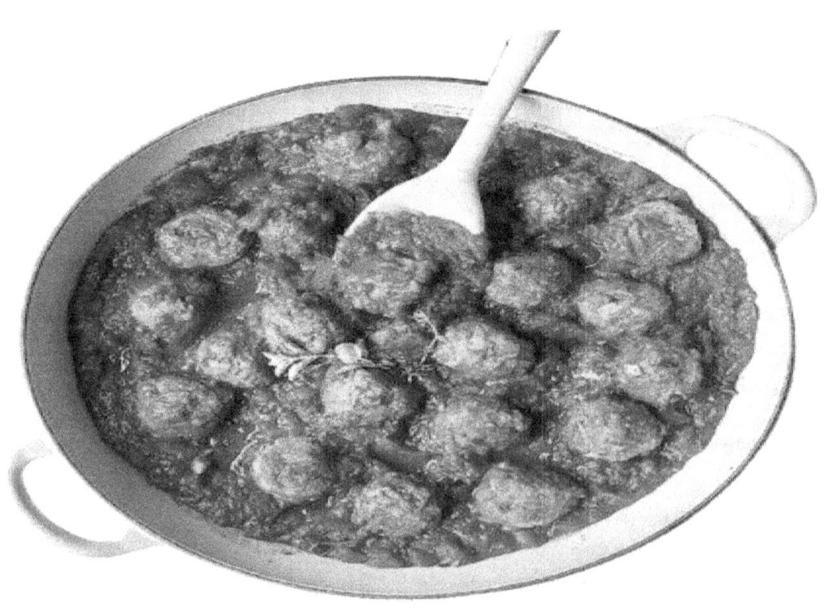

INTRODUCTION

Hello there, fellow food enthusiast! I'm Lorene Peachey, your go-to nutritionist, and I'm thrilled to share my journey with you through the tantalizing world of gluten-free slow cooking. Welcome to a realm where flavour knows no bounds, and health takes centre stage. But before we dive into the delectable recipes that await you in this cookbook, let me take you on a heartwarming journey that started with – the lovely Charlotte Applewood.

Charlotte, a vibrant soul with a zest for life, came to me with a culinary conundrum that echoed the struggles of many. She had traversed through various cookbooks, desperately seeking a gluten-free haven that would satiate her taste buds and nourish her body. The gluten-free path, though promising, often felt like a maze without a solution. Charlotte had faced disappointment after disappointment, and it seemed like her quest for a satisfying, gluten-free meal was destined to be an elusive one.

That's when she stumbled upon my cookbook. Imagine the joy and relief that twinkled in her eyes when she discovered a treasure trove of recipes that not only catered to her gluten-free needs but also celebrated the art of slow cooking. It wasn't just about the ingredients; it was about crafting an experience, a journey through comforting aromas and mouthwatering Flavors that danced on her palate.

As Charlotte shared her newfound joy, she articulated something that resonated deeply with me: "Finally, a cookbook that doesn't just tell me what to eat but makes me fall in love with the process."

But why the fuss about gluten-free, you might ask? Well, beyond being the latest health trend, gluten-free living has profound benefits that extend beyond the physical. It's about nourishing your body and soul, embracing flavors that ignite your senses, and fostering a lifestyle that radiates well-being. Gluten-free isn't just a diet; it's a journey toward feeling your absolute best.

Consider this: when was the last time you truly relished a meal without the nagging aftermath of discomfort? Picture a world where digestion is seamless, energy levels soar, and the joy of eating is uncompromised. Gluten-free living is your ticket to that world – a world where your body thanks you for every bite.

Now, let's talk about the not-so-pleasant side of the culinary world – the dangers lurking in unhealthy eating. It's a reality we often overlook in our fast-paced lives. Processed foods, laden with gluten and other harmful additives, may provide momentary pleasure, but at what cost? The long-term consequences can be dire, ranging from digestive issues to chronic illnesses that mar the quality of life.

Here's where the magic of gluten-free slow cooking steps in. It's not just about avoiding gluten; it's about embracing a lifestyle that prioritizes fresh, wholesome ingredients. My cookbook doesn't just offer recipes; it extends a helping hand toward a healthier, happier you.

So, what makes this cookbook different? It's more than just a collection of recipes; it's a culinary companion on your journey to wellness. The advantages are aplenty. You'll discover the joy of savouring rich, flavourful dishes without compromising your health. With each recipe, you're not just cooking; you're creating an experience, a moment to relish and share with loved ones.

Let's flip the narrative. Imagine your kitchen becoming a haven of health, where the sizzle of a slow-cooked meal mirrors the vibrancy of your well-being. Envision a future where you don't just eat to survive but relish every bite, knowing it fuels your body with the nutrients it deserves.

As you embark on this gluten-free journey, ask yourself: How does your current diet make you feel? Are you tired of the monotony and the aftermath of guilt that accompanies unhealthy choices? Are you ready to embrace a lifestyle that transcends diets and becomes a celebration of good food, good health, and good living?

My dear reader, the power to transform your culinary world lies at your fingertips. This cookbook is your ally, your guide to a gluten-free haven where taste knows no compromise. It's time to bid farewell to culinary frustrations and welcome a life where every meal is a step toward your best self.

So, are you ready to embark on this flavourful journey with me? Let the aroma of wholesome ingredients fill your kitchen and let the sizzle of slow cooking be the soundtrack of your newfound culinary adventure. Together, let's redefine the way we eat and live, one gluten-free, slow-cooked masterpiece at a time. Cheers to a healthier, happier you!

Contact the Author

Thank you for reading my book! I would love to hear from you, whether you have feedback, questions, or just want to share your thoughts. Your feedback means a lot to me and helps me improve as a writer.

Please don't hesitate to reach out to me through

lorenepeachey@gmail.com

I look forward to connecting with my readers and appreciate your support in this literary journey. Your thoughts and comments are valuable to me.

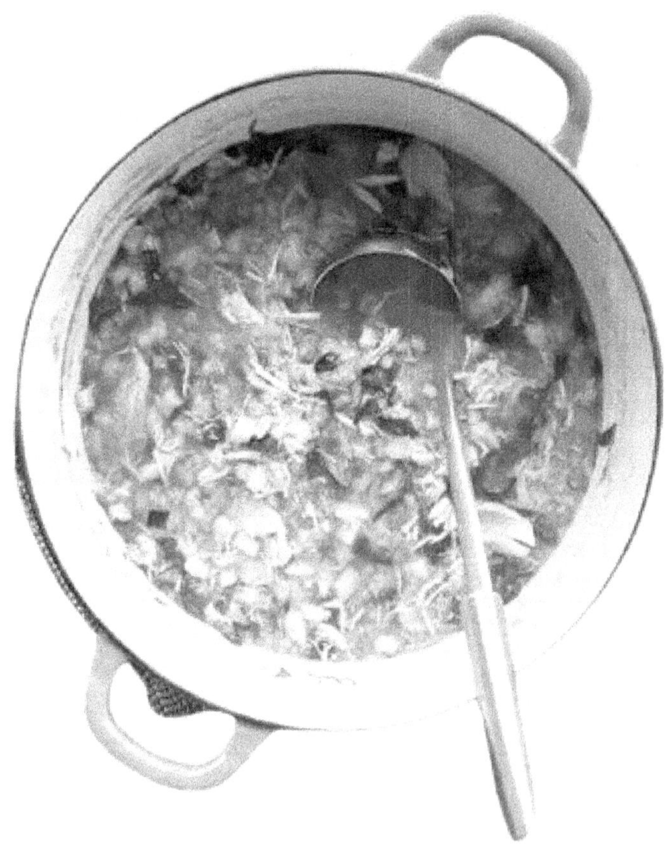

CHAPTER 1

UNDERSTANDING GLUTEN-FREE COOKING

Gluten-free cooking has gained popularity due to the increasing awareness of gluten-related sensitivities and conditions, such as celiac disease. Gluten is a protein found in wheat, barley, rye, and their derivatives. People with gluten sensitivities must adhere to a gluten-free diet to avoid adverse health effects. Gluten-free cooking involves using alternative flours and ingredients to create delicious and safe meals for those with gluten intolerance.

Benefits of Slow Cooking for Gluten-Free Meals

Slow cooking is a versatile and convenient method that can enhance the flavors and textures of gluten-free meals. Here are some benefits of incorporating slow cooking into your gluten-free cooking routine:

Tenderizes Tough Cuts of Meat: Slow cooking is excellent for breaking down the collagen in tougher cuts of meat, resulting in tender and flavorful dishes without the need for gluten-containing marinades or sauces.

Enhanced Flavor Development: The slow cooking process allows flavors to meld and intensify, creating rich and savory gluten-free dishes. This is particularly beneficial when using a variety of herbs, spices, and gluten-free broths.

Convenience and Timesaving: Slow cookers are time-saving kitchen tools that require minimal hands-on effort. This is especially useful for individuals with gluten sensitivities who may need to invest more time in ingredient sourcing and label reading.

One-Pot Wonders: Slow cookers are ideal for creating one-pot meals, reducing the need for multiple pots and pans. This simplifies the cooking process and minimizes the risk of cross-contamination with gluten-containing ingredients.

Essential Ingredients for Gluten-Free Cooking

Gluten-Free Flours: Use alternative flours such as rice flour, almond flour, coconut flour, or a gluten-free flour blend in place of wheat flour in recipes.

Gluten-Free Grains: Incorporate gluten-free grains like quinoa, millet, buckwheat, and certified gluten-free oats into your meals.

Fresh Fruits and Vegetables: Focus on incorporating a variety of fresh, whole fruits and vegetables to add nutritional value and flavor to your gluten-free dishes.

Gluten-Free Condiments and Sauces: Check labels to ensure that condiments and sauces are gluten-free. Opt for gluten-free soy sauce or tamari, and choose condiments without hidden gluten additives.

Kitchen Tools for Gluten-Free Cooking

Dedicated Gluten-Free Utensils: To prevent cross-contamination, consider having separate cutting boards, utensils, and kitchen equipment specifically designated for gluten-free cooking.

Quality Gluten-Free Cookware: Invest in non-stick or stainless-steel cookware to avoid the risk of gluten contamination from scratched or porous surfaces.

Food Processor or Blender: These tools are essential for creating gluten-free flours from whole grains or nuts, expanding your options for gluten-free baking.

CHAPTER 2

GLUTEN-FREE BASICS

Adopting a gluten-free lifestyle involves eliminating foods containing gluten—a protein found in wheat, barley, rye, and their derivatives. This dietary choice is essential for individuals with celiac disease, gluten sensitivity, or those aiming for a gluten-free diet. Mastering gluten-free basics is the key to creating delicious and safe meals. Here's a guide to understanding and navigating gluten-free cooking:

Gluten-Free Flours and Alternatives

Almond Flour: Ground from almonds, almond flour adds a nutty richness to baked goods.

Coconut Flour: Made from dried coconut, it's high in fiber and imparts a subtle coconut flavor.

Rice Flour: A versatile option with a mild taste, both white and brown rice flour are commonly used.

Quinoa Flour: Ground from quinoa seeds, it offers a unique flavor and nutritional benefits.

Buckwheat Flour: Despite its name, buckwheat is gluten-free and brings a robust flavor to recipes.

Cornmeal: Ideal for a variety of dishes, including cornbread and coating for frying.

Tapioca Flour/Starch: A light, starchy flour commonly used in gluten-free baking.

Sorghum Flour: With a mild taste, sorghum flour is often used in gluten-free blends.

Creating Gluten-Free Blends

Crafting your gluten-free flour blend allows you to customize the texture and flavor of your baked goods. Here's a simple all-purpose gluten-free flour blend:

All-Purpose Gluten-Free Flour Blend:

- ✓ 1 cup white rice flour
- ✓ 1 cup brown rice flour
- ✓ 1 cup potato starch
- ✓ 1/2 cup tapioca flour/starch
- ✓ 1/2 cup sorghum flour or millet flour

Combine these flours thoroughly and use as a one-to-one substitute for all-purpose wheat flour in various recipes.

Tips for Gluten-Free Baking in a Slow Cooker

Select the Right Pan: Choose a heat-resistant and oven-safe pan that fits inside your slow cooker. Non-stick or silicone pans work well.

Line the Pan: Prevent sticking and ease removal by lining the pan with parchment paper.

Check Doneness: Gluten-free baked goods may require more or less time than traditional recipes. Use a toothpick to check for doneness and adjust cooking time accordingly.

Manage Moisture: Gluten-free flours can absorb more moisture. Adjust the batter consistency as needed, adding extra liquid or reducing cooking time to prevent dryness.

CHAPTER 3

BREAKFAST DELIGHTS

Quinoa Breakfast Porridge

Cooking Time: 4 hours on low

Serving: 4

Ingredients:

- ✓ 1 cup quinoa, rinsed
- ✓ 2 cups almond milk
- ✓ 1/4 cup maple syrup
- ✓ 1 teaspoon cinnamon
- ✓ 1/2 cup chopped nuts and fresh berries for topping

Instructions:

1. Combine quinoa, almond milk, maple syrup, and cinnamon in the slow cooker.
2. Cook on low for 4 hours.
3. Serve topped with nuts and berries.

Nutritional Information: 250 calories, 45g carbs, 8g protein, 5g fat, 6g fiber.

Slow Cooker Omelets Casserole

Cooking Time: 3 hours on low

Serving: 6

Ingredients:

- ✓ 8 eggs, beaten
- ✓ 1 cup diced vegetables (bell peppers, spinach, tomatoes)
- ✓ 1 cup cooked and crumbled turkey sausage
- ✓ 1 cup shredded cheese
- ✓ Salt and pepper to taste

Instructions:

1. Whisk eggs and combine with vegetables, sausage, cheese, salt, and pepper.
2. Pour mixture into the slow cooker.
3. Cook on low for 3 hours.

Nutritional Information: 220 calories, 5g carbs, 15g protein, 16g fat, 2g fiber.

Cinnamon Apple Steel-Cut Oats

Cooking Time: 6 hours on low

Serving: 6

Ingredients:

- ✓ 2 cups steel-cut oats
- ✓ 4 cups unsweetened almond milk
- ✓ 2 apples, peeled and diced
- ✓ 1/4 cup honey
- ✓ 1 teaspoon cinnamon

Instructions:

1. Combine oats, almond milk, apples, honey, and cinnamon in the slow cooker.
2. Cook on low for 6 hours.
3. Stir well before serving.

Nutritional Information: 280 calories, 50g carbs, 8g protein, 5g fat, 8g fiber.

Sweet Potato and Sausage Breakfast Casserole

Cooking Time: 4 hours on low

Serving: 8

Ingredients:

- ✓ 2 sweet potatoes, peeled and grated
- ✓ 1 pound turkey sausage, cooked and crumbled
- ✓ 1 cup spinach, chopped
- ✓ 8 eggs, beaten
- ✓ 1 cup unsweetened almond milk

Instructions:

1. Layer sweet potatoes, sausage, and spinach in the slow cooker.
2. Whisk together eggs and almond milk, pour over the layers.
3. Cook on low for 4 hours.

Nutritional Information: 280 calories, 20g carbs, 18g protein, 14g fat, 4g fiber.

Banana Nut Quinoa Porridge

Cooking Time: 3 hours on low

Serving: 4

Ingredients:

- ✓ 1 cup quinoa, rinsed
- ✓ 2 cups coconut milk
- ✓ 2 ripe bananas, mashed
- ✓ 1/2 cup chopped nuts
- ✓ 1 teaspoon vanilla extract

Instructions:

1. Combine quinoa, coconut milk, bananas, nuts, and vanilla in the slow cooker.
2. Cook on low for 3 hours.
3. Serve warm.

Nutritional Information: 300 calories, 40g carbs, 8g protein, 12g fat, 5g fiber.

Blueberry Lemon Chia Pudding

Cooking Time: 2 hours on low

Serving: 4

Ingredients:

- ✓ 1/2 cup chia seeds
- ✓ 2 cups unsweetened almond milk
- ✓ 1 cup blueberries (fresh or frozen)
- ✓ Zest of 1 lemon
- ✓ 2 tablespoons maple syrup

Instructions:

1. Mix chia seeds, almond milk, blueberries, lemon zest, and maple syrup in the slow cooker.
2. Cook on low for 2 hours, stirring occasionally.
3. Chill before serving.

Nutritional Information: 180 calories, 20g carbs, 5g protein, 10g fat, 8g fiber.

Pumpkin Spice Oatmeal

Cooking Time: 4 hours on low

Serving: 6

Ingredients:

- ✓ 2 cups old-fashioned oats
- ✓ 4 cups almond milk
- ✓ 1 cup canned pumpkin puree
- ✓ 1/4 cup maple syrup
- ✓ 1 teaspoon pumpkin spice blend

Instructions:

1. Combine oats, almond milk, pumpkin puree, maple syrup, and pumpkin spice in the slow cooker.
2. Cook on low for 4 hours.
3. Stir well before serving.

Nutritional Information: 240 calories, 40g carbs, 6g protein, 6g fat, 5g fiber.

Coconut-Berry Breakfast Quinoa

Cooking Time: 3 hours on low

Serving: 4

Ingredients:

- ✓ 1 cup quinoa, rinsed
- ✓ 2 cups coconut milk
- ✓ 1 cup mixed berries (strawberries, blueberries, raspberries)
- ✓ 1/4 cup shredded coconut
- ✓ 2 tablespoons honey

Instructions:

1. Combine quinoa, coconut milk, berries, shredded coconut, and honey in the slow cooker.
2. Cook on low for 3 hours.
3. Top with extra berries before serving.

Nutritional Information: 280 calories, 35g carbs, 6g protein, 12g fat, 5g fiber.

Apple Cinnamon Breakfast Risotto

Cooking Time: 3 hours on low

Serving: 6

Ingredients:

- ✓ 1 cup Arborio rice
- ✓ 2 apples, peeled and diced
- ✓ 4 cups unsweetened almond milk
- ✓ 1/4 cup maple syrup
- ✓ 1 teaspoon cinnamon

Instructions:

1. Combine rice, apples, almond milk, maple syrup, and cinnamon in the slow cooker.
2. Cook on low for 3 hours, stirring occasionally.
3. Serve warm.

Nutritional Information: 220 calories, 45g carbs, 5g protein, 3g fat, 4g fiber.

Cherry Almond Breakfast Quinoa

Cooking Time: 2.5 hours on low

Serving: 4

Ingredients:

- ✓ 1 cup quinoa, rinsed
- ✓ 2 cups almond milk
- ✓ 1 cup cherries, pitted and halved
- ✓ 1/4 cup chopped almonds
- ✓ 2 tablespoons honey

Instructions:

1. Combine quinoa, almond milk, cherries, almonds, and honey in the slow cooker.
2. Cook on low for 2.5 hours.
3. Drizzle with additional honey before serving.

Nutritional Information: 260 calories, 35g carbs, 8g protein, 10g fat, 5g fiber.

CHAPTER 4

HEARTY SOUPS AND STEWS

Chicken and Vegetable Quinoa Soup

Cooking Time: 4 hours on low

Serving: 6

Ingredients:

- ✓ 1 lb boneless, skinless chicken thighs, diced
- ✓ 1 cup quinoa, rinsed
- ✓ 4 cups chicken broth
- ✓ 2 carrots, sliced
- ✓ 1 cup kale, chopped

Instructions:

1. Combine chicken, quinoa, broth, carrots, and kale in the slow cooker.
2. Cook on low for 4 hours.
3. Shred chicken before serving.

Nutritional Information: 280 calories, 25g carbs, 25g protein, 8g fat, 5g fiber.

Beef and Sweet Potato Stew

Cooking Time: 6 hours on low

Serving: 8

Ingredients:

- ✓ 2 lbs beef stew meat, cubed
- ✓ 2 sweet potatoes, peeled and diced
- ✓ 1 onion, chopped
- ✓ 4 cups beef broth
- ✓ 1 cup green beans, trimmed

Instructions:

1. Combine beef, sweet potatoes, onion, broth, and green beans in the slow cooker.
2. Cook on low for 6 hours.
3. Season with salt and pepper before serving.

Nutritional Information: 350 calories, 30g carbs, 35g protein, 10g fat, 6g fiber.

Lentil and Vegetable Soup

Cooking Time: 5 hours on low

Serving: 6

Ingredients:

- ✓ 1 cup dry green lentils, rinsed
- ✓ 1 onion, diced
- ✓ 3 carrots, sliced
- ✓ 3 celery stalks, chopped
- ✓ 4 cups vegetable broth

Instructions:

1. Combine lentils, onion, carrots, celery, and broth in the slow cooker.
2. Cook on low for 5 hours.
3. Season with herbs and salt to taste.

Nutritional Information: 240 calories, 40g carbs, 15g protein, 2g fat, 10g fiber.

Turkey and Butternut Squash Chili

Cooking Time: 4 hours on low

Serving: 8

Ingredients:

- ✓ 1 lb ground turkey
- ✓ 2 cups butternut squash, diced
- ✓ 1 can black beans, drained and rinsed
- ✓ 1 can diced tomatoes
- ✓ 2 tablespoons chili powder

Instructions:

1. Brown turkey in a pan, then combine with squash, black beans, tomatoes, and chili powder in the slow cooker.
2. Cook on low for 4 hours.
3. Garnish with cilantro and shredded cheese before serving.

Nutritional Information: 290 calories, 30g carbs, 25g protein, 8g fat, 8g fiber.

Italian Sausage and Vegetable Soup

Cooking Time: 3 hours on low

Serving: 6

Ingredients:

- ✓ 1 lb gluten-free Italian sausage, sliced
- ✓ 2 zucchinis, diced
- ✓ 1 bell pepper, chopped
- ✓ 1 can diced tomatoes
- ✓ 4 cups chicken broth

Instructions:

1. Combine sausage, zucchinis, bell pepper, tomatoes, and broth in the slow cooker.
2. Cook on low for 3 hours.
3. Serve with a sprinkle of grated Parmesan.

Nutritional Information: 320 calories, 15g carbs, 20g protein, 22g fat, 5g fiber.

Mushroom and Wild Rice Stew

Cooking Time: 5 hours on low

Serving: 6

Ingredients:

- ✓ 1 cup wild rice, rinsed
- ✓ 1 lb mushrooms, sliced
- ✓ 1 onion, diced
- ✓ 3 cloves garlic, minced
- ✓ 4 cups vegetable broth

Instructions:

1. Combine rice, mushrooms, onion, garlic, and broth in the slow cooker.
2. Cook on low for 5 hours.
3. Stir in a splash of balsamic vinegar before serving.

Nutritional Information: 260 calories, 45g carbs, 8g protein, 5g fat, 6g fiber.

Salmon and Corn Chowder

Cooking Time: 4 hours on low

Serving: 4

Ingredients:

- ✓ 1 lb salmon fillets, diced
- ✓ 2 cups corn kernels (fresh or frozen)
- ✓ 1 potato, peeled and diced
- ✓ 2 cups coconut milk
- ✓ 2 cups fish or vegetable broth

Instructions:

1. Combine salmon, corn, potato, coconut milk, and broth in the slow cooker.
2. Cook on low for 4 hours.
3. Season with dill and salt before serving.

Nutritional Information: 320 calories, 30g carbs, 25g protein, 15g fat, 4g fiber.

Vegetarian Chili with Quinoa

Cooking Time: 3.5 hours on low

Serving: 6

Ingredients:

- ✓ 1 cup quinoa, rinsed
- ✓ 1 can kidney beans, drained and rinsed
- ✓ 1 can black beans, drained and rinsed
- ✓ 1 can diced tomatoes
- ✓ 1 bell pepper, chopped

Instructions:

1. Combine quinoa, beans, tomatoes, and bell pepper in the slow cooker.
2. Cook on low for 3.5 hours.
3. Top with avocado and cilantro before serving.

Nutritional Information: 280 calories, 45g carbs, 12g protein, 5g fat, 10g fiber.

Thai Coconut Chicken Soup

Cooking Time: 4 hours on low

Serving: 4

Ingredients:

- ✓ 1 lb chicken breast, thinly sliced
- ✓ 2 cups sliced mushrooms
- ✓ 1 can coconut milk
- ✓ 2 cups chicken broth
- ✓ 1 tablespoon red curry paste

Instructions:

1. Combine chicken, mushrooms, coconut milk, broth, and curry paste in the slow cooker.
2. Cook on low for 4 hours.
3. Stir in lime juice and cilantro before serving.

Nutritional Information: 310 calories, 10g carbs, 30g protein, 18g fat, 3g fiber.

Root Vegetable and Lentil Stew

Cooking Time: 5 hours on low

Serving: 6

Ingredients:

- ✓ 1 cup dry brown lentils, rinsed
- ✓ 2 carrots, peeled and chopped
- ✓ 2 parsnips, peeled and chopped
- ✓ 1 sweet potato, peeled and diced
- ✓ 4 cups vegetable broth

Instructions:

1. Combine lentils, carrots, parsnips, sweet potato, and broth in the slow cooker.
2. Cook on low for 5 hours.
3. Season with thyme and salt before serving.

Nutritional Information: 240 calories, 45g carbs, 12g protein, 2g fat, 10g fiber.

CHAPER 5

TENDER MEATS

Balsamic Glazed Chicken

Cooking Time: 4 hours on low

Serving: 4

Ingredients:

- ✓ 4 boneless, skinless chicken breasts
- ✓ 1/2 cup balsamic vinegar
- ✓ 1/4 cup honey
- ✓ 2 cloves garlic, minced
- ✓ 1 teaspoon dried thyme

Instructions:

1. Place chicken breasts in the slow cooker.
2. Mix balsamic vinegar, honey, garlic, and thyme; pour over chicken.
3. Cook on low for 4 hours.

Nutritional Information: 320 calories, 15g carbs, 30g protein, 10g fat, 0g fiber.

Tender Pork Carnitas

Cooking Time: 6 hours on low

Serving: 8

Ingredients:

- ✓ 3 lbs pork shoulder, cut into chunks
- ✓ 1 onion, sliced
- ✓ 4 cloves garlic, minced
- ✓ 1 teaspoon cumin
- ✓ 1 teaspoon oregano

Instructions:

1. Combine pork, onion, garlic, cumin, and oregano in the slow cooker.
2. Cook on low for 6 hours.
3. Shred pork and broil for crispy edges before serving.

Nutritional Information: 280 calories, 2g carbs, 25g protein, 20g fat, 1g fiber.

Maple-Dijon Glazed Salmon

Cooking Time: 2.5 hours on low

Serving: 4

Ingredients:

- ✓ 4 salmon fillets
- ✓ 1/4 cup maple syrup
- ✓ 2 tablespoons Dijon mustard
- ✓ 1 tablespoon soy sauce (gluten-free)
- ✓ 1 teaspoon garlic powder

Instructions:

1. Place salmon fillets in the slow cooker.
2. Whisk together maple syrup, Dijon mustard, soy sauce, and garlic powder; pour over salmon.
3. Cook on low for 2.5 hours.

Nutritional Information: 300 calories, 15g carbs, 25g protein, 15g fat, 0g fiber.

Italian Herb Beef Roast

Cooking Time: 5 hours on low

Serving: 6

Ingredients:

- ✓ 2.5 lbs beef chuck roast
- ✓ 1 cup beef broth
- ✓ 1/4 cup tomato paste
- ✓ 2 teaspoons dried Italian herbs
- ✓ Salt and pepper to taste

Instructions:

1. Place beef roast in the slow cooker.
2. Mix beef broth, tomato paste, Italian herbs, salt, and pepper; pour over the roast.
3. Cook on low for 5 hours.

Nutritional Information: 350 calories, 4g carbs, 35g protein, 22g fat, 1g fiber.

Honey Garlic Turkey Breast

Cooking Time: 4 hours on low

Serving: 6

Ingredients:

- ✓ 3 lbs turkey breast
- ✓ 1/3 cup honey
- ✓ 1/4 cup gluten-free soy sauce
- ✓ 3 cloves garlic, minced
- ✓ 1 teaspoon dried rosemary

Instructions:

1. Place turkey breast in the slow cooker.
2. Mix honey, soy sauce, garlic, and rosemary; pour over the turkey.
3. Cook on low for 4 hours.

Nutritional Information: 280 calories, 10g carbs, 35g protein, 10g fat, 0g fiber.

Lemon Herb Lamb Chops

Cooking Time: 3 hours on low

Serving: 4

Ingredients:

- ✓ 8 lamb chops
- ✓ 1/4 cup olive oil
- ✓ Juice of 2 lemons
- ✓ 2 teaspoons dried thyme
- ✓ Salt and pepper to taste

Instructions:

1. Place lamb chops in the slow cooker.
2. Mix olive oil, lemon juice, thyme, salt, and pepper; pour over lamb chops.
3. Cook on low for 3 hours.

Nutritional Information: 380 calories, 2g carbs, 30g protein, 28g fat, 0g fiber.

Spicy BBQ Pulled Chicken

Cooking Time: 4 hours on low

Serving: 8

Ingredients:

- ✓ 2 lbs boneless, skinless chicken thighs
- ✓ 1 cup gluten-free BBQ sauce
- ✓ 1/4 cup apple cider vinegar
- ✓ 2 tablespoons honey
- ✓ 1 teaspoon smoked paprika

Instructions:

1. Place chicken thighs in the slow cooker.
2. Mix BBQ sauce, apple cider vinegar, honey, and smoked paprika; pour over chicken.
3. Cook on low for 4 hours.

Nutritional Information: 290 calories, 20g carbs, 30g protein, 10g fat, 0g fiber.

Herbed Turkey Meatballs

Cooking Time: 3 hours on low

Serving: 6

Ingredients:

- ✓ 1.5 lbs ground turkey
- ✓ 1/2 cup gluten-free breadcrumbs
- ✓ 1/4 cup grated Parmesan cheese
- ✓ 2 teaspoons dried Italian herbs
- ✓ 1 egg

Instructions:

1. Mix ground turkey, breadcrumbs, Parmesan, Italian herbs, and egg.
2. Form meatballs and place them in the slow cooker.
3. Cook on low for 3 hours.

Nutritional Information: 220 calories, 5g carbs, 25g protein, 12g fat, 0g fiber.

Coconut Lime Shrimp Curry

Cooking Time: 2 hours on low

Serving: 4

Ingredients:

- ✓ 1 lb large shrimp, peeled and deveined
- ✓ 1 can coconut milk
- ✓ Juice of 2 limes
- ✓ 2 tablespoons red curry paste
- ✓ 1 tablespoon fish sauce (gluten-free)

Instructions:

1. Place shrimp in the slow cooker.
2. Mix coconut milk, lime juice, red curry paste, and fish sauce; pour over shrimp.
3. Cook on low for 2 hours.

Nutritional Information: 260 calories, 8g carbs, 20g protein, 16g fat, 1g fiber.

Teriyaki Pineapple Chicken

Cooking Time: 4 hours on low

Serving: 6

Ingredients:

- ✓ 2 lbs boneless, skinless chicken thighs
- ✓ 1 cup gluten-free teriyaki sauce
- ✓ 1 can pineapple chunks, drained
- ✓ 1/4 cup chopped green onions
- ✓ 1 teaspoon sesame seeds

Instructions:

1. Place chicken thighs in the slow cooker.
2. Mix teriyaki sauce and pineapple chunks; pour over chicken.
3. Cook on low for 4 hours.
4. Garnish with green onions and sesame seeds before serving.

Nutritional Information: 320 calories, 20g carbs, 30g protein, 12g fat, 1g fiber.

CHAPTER 6

VEGETARIAN WONDERS

Slow Cooker Lentil Soup

Cooking Time: 4 hours on low

Serving: 6

Ingredients:

- ✓ 1 cup dry green lentils, rinsed
- ✓ 1 onion, diced
- ✓ 3 carrots, sliced
- ✓ 3 celery stalks, chopped
- ✓ 4 cups vegetable broth

Instructions:

1. Combine lentils, onion, carrots, celery, and broth in the slow cooker.
2. Cook on low for 4 hours.
3. Season with herbs and salt to taste.

Nutritional Information: 240 calories, 40g carbs, 15g protein, 2g fat, 10g fiber.

Quinoa and Black Bean Stuffed Peppers

Cooking Time: 3.5 hours on low

Serving: 4

Ingredients:

- ✓ 4 bell peppers, halved and seeds removed
- ✓ 1 cup cooked quinoa
- ✓ 1 can black beans, drained and rinsed
- ✓ 1 cup corn kernels (fresh or frozen)
- ✓ 1 cup salsa

Instructions:

1. Fill each pepper half with a mixture of quinoa, black beans, corn, and salsa.
2. Arrange in the slow cooker and cook on low for 3.5 hours.
3. Top with cheese before serving, if desired.

Nutritional Information: 280 calories, 50g carbs, 12g protein, 5g fat, 10g fiber.

Vegetarian Tikka Masala

Cooking Time: 4 hours on low

Serving: 4

Ingredients:

- ✓ 2 cups cauliflower florets
- ✓ 1 can chickpeas, drained and rinsed
- ✓ 1 onion, finely chopped
- ✓ 2 cups tomato sauce
- ✓ 1/2 cup coconut milk

Instructions:

1. Combine cauliflower, chickpeas, onion, tomato sauce, and coconut milk in the slow cooker.
2. Cook on low for 4 hours.
3. Serve over rice or with naan bread.

Nutritional Information: 320 calories, 40g carbs, 10g protein, 15g fat, 8g fiber.

Sweet Potato and Chickpea Curry

Cooking Time: 3 hours on low

Serving: 6

Ingredients:

- ✓ 2 sweet potatoes, peeled and diced
- ✓ 1 can chickpeas, drained and rinsed
- ✓ 1 onion, chopped
- ✓ 2 cups vegetable broth
- ✓ 1 can coconut milk

Instructions:

1. Combine sweet potatoes, chickpeas, onion, broth, and coconut milk in the slow cooker.
2. Cook on low for 3 hours.
3. Stir in spinach before serving.

Nutritional Information: 280 calories, 40g carbs, 8g protein, 10g fat, 8g fiber.

Mushroom and Spinach Risotto

Cooking Time: 2.5 hours on low

Serving: 4

Ingredients:

- ✓ 1 cup Arborio rice
- ✓ 2 cups mushrooms, sliced
- ✓ 1 onion, finely chopped
- ✓ 4 cups vegetable broth
- ✓ 1 cup fresh spinach

Instructions:

1. Combine rice, mushrooms, onion, broth, and spinach in the slow cooker.
2. Cook on low for 2.5 hours, stirring occasionally.
3. Finish with a sprinkle of Parmesan cheese before serving.

Nutritional Information: 300 calories, 50g carbs, 8g protein, 5g fat, 6g fiber.

Butternut Squash and Coconut Soup

Cooking Time: 4 hours on low

Serving: 6

Ingredients:

- ✓ 1 butternut squash, peeled and diced
- ✓ 1 onion, chopped
- ✓ 2 cloves garlic, minced
- ✓ 4 cups vegetable broth
- ✓ 1 can coconut milk

Instructions:

1. Combine butternut squash, onion, garlic, broth, and coconut milk in the slow cooker.
2. Cook on low for 4 hours.
3. Blend until smooth before serving.

Nutritional Information: 220 calories, 30g carbs, 3g protein, 12g fat, 6g fiber.

Eggplant and Tomato Casserole

Cooking Time: 3 hours on low

Serving: 6

Ingredients:

- ✓ 2 eggplants, sliced
- ✓ 2 cups cherry tomatoes, halved
- ✓ 1 onion, sliced
- ✓ 2 cloves garlic, minced
- ✓ 1 can diced tomatoes

Instructions:

1. Layer eggplants, cherry tomatoes, onion, garlic, and canned tomatoes in the slow cooker.
2. Cook on low for 3 hours.
3. Top with fresh basil before serving.

Nutritional Information: 180 calories, 40g carbs, 5g protein, 2g fat, 10g fiber.

Chickpea and Vegetable Tagine

Cooking Time: 4 hours on low

Serving: 4

Ingredients:

- ✓ 2 cans chickpeas, drained and rinsed
- ✓ 2 carrots, sliced
- ✓ 1 zucchini, diced
- ✓ 1 onion, chopped
- ✓ 2 cups vegetable broth

Instructions:

1. Combine chickpeas, carrots, zucchini, onion, and broth in the slow cooker.
2. Cook on low for 4 hours.
3. Stir in chopped apricots before serving.

Nutritional Information: 260 calories, 45g carbs, 12g protein, 5g fat, 10g fiber.

Mexican Quinoa Casserole

Cooking Time: 3 hours on low

Serving: 6

Ingredients:

- ✓ 1 cup quinoa, rinsed
- ✓ 1 can black beans, drained and rinsed
- ✓ 1 cup corn kernels (fresh or frozen)
- ✓ 1 bell pepper, diced
- ✓ 2 cups salsa

Instructions:

1. Combine quinoa, black beans, corn, bell pepper, and salsa in the slow cooker.
2. Cook on low for 3 hours.
3. Top with avocado and cilantro before serving.

Nutritional Information: 280 calories, 50g carbs, 10g protein, 5g fat, 8g fiber.

Vegetarian Chili with Sweet Potatoes

Cooking Time: 4 hours on low

Serving: 8

Ingredients:

- ✓ 2 sweet potatoes, peeled and diced
- ✓ 1 can kidney beans, drained and rinsed
- ✓ 1 can black beans, drained and rinsed
- ✓ 1 can diced tomatoes
- ✓ 1 onion, chopped

Instructions:

1. Combine sweet potatoes, kidney beans, black beans, tomatoes, and onion in the slow cooker.
2. Cook on low for 4 hours.
3. Season with chili powder and cumin before serving.

Nutritional Information: 240 calories, 45g carbs, 10g protein, 2g fat, 8g fiber.

CHAPTER 7

SIDES AND SNACKS

Cinnamon Maple Glazed Carrots

Cooking Time: 2 hours on low

Serving: 4

Ingredients:

- ✓ 1 lb baby carrots
- ✓ 2 tablespoons maple syrup
- ✓ 1 tablespoon melted coconut oil
- ✓ 1 teaspoon ground cinnamon

Instructions:

1. Toss carrots in maple syrup, coconut oil, and cinnamon.
2. Place in the slow cooker and cook on low for 2 hours.
3. Garnish with fresh parsley before serving.

Nutritional Information: 120 calories, 20g carbs, 1g protein, 5g fat, 4g fiber.

Garlic Herb Mashed Potatoes

Cooking Time: 3 hours on low

Serving: 6

Ingredients:

- ✓ 2 lbs potatoes, peeled and diced
- ✓ 4 cloves garlic, minced
- ✓ 1/2 cup vegetable broth
- ✓ 1/4 cup dairy-free butter

Instructions:

1. Combine potatoes, garlic, broth, and butter in the slow cooker.
2. Cook on low for 3 hours, then mash.
3. Season with salt and pepper before serving.

Nutritional Information: 180 calories, 35g carbs, 2g protein, 5g fat, 4g fiber.

Rosemary Parmesan Polenta

Cooking Time: 2.5 hours on low

Serving: 4

Ingredients:

- ✓ 1 cup cornmeal
- ✓ 4 cups vegetable broth
- ✓ 1/2 cup grated Parmesan cheese
- ✓ 2 tablespoons chopped fresh rosemary

Instructions:

1. Whisk cornmeal, broth, Parmesan, and rosemary in the slow cooker.
2. Cook on low for 2.5 hours, stirring occasionally.
3. Serve as a creamy side dish.

Nutritional Information: 220 calories, 30g carbs, 8g protein, 8g fat, 3g fiber.

Maple Dijon Brussels Sprouts

Cooking Time: 2 hours on low

Serving: 4

Ingredients:

- ✓ 1 lb Brussels sprouts, trimmed and halved
- ✓ 2 tablespoons maple syrup
- ✓ 1 tablespoon Dijon mustard
- ✓ 2 tablespoons olive oil

Instructions:

1. Toss Brussels sprouts in maple syrup, Dijon, and olive oil.
2. Place in the slow cooker and cook on low for 2 hours.
3. Sprinkle with sea salt before serving.

Nutritional Information: 150 calories, 20g carbs, 4g protein, 7g fat, 5g fiber.

Quinoa and Vegetable Stuffed Peppers

Cooking Time: 3.5 hours on low

Serving: 6

Ingredients:

- ✓ 6 bell peppers, halved and seeds removed
- ✓ 1 cup cooked quinoa
- ✓ 1 zucchini, diced
- ✓ 1 cup cherry tomatoes, halved

Instructions:

1. Fill each pepper half with a mixture of quinoa, zucchini, and tomatoes.
2. Arrange in the slow cooker and cook on low for 3.5 hours.
3. Top with fresh basil before serving.

Nutritional Information: 180 calories, 30g carbs, 6g protein, 5g fat, 5g fiber.

Cranberry Orange Sauce

Cooking Time: 2 hours on low

Serving: 8

Ingredients:

- ✓ 2 cups fresh cranberries
- ✓ 1/2 cup orange juice
- ✓ 1/2 cup maple syrup
- ✓ Zest of 1 orange

Instructions:

1. Combine cranberries, orange juice, maple syrup, and orange zest in the slow cooker.
2. Cook on low for 2 hours, stirring occasionally.
3. Serve as a flavorful sauce for Thanksgiving or any occasion.

Nutritional Information: 100 calories, 25g carbs, 0g protein, 0g fat, 3g fiber.

Curry Roasted Cauliflower

Cooking Time: 2.5 hours on low

Serving: 4

Ingredients:

- ✓ 1 head cauliflower, cut into florets
- ✓ 2 tablespoons olive oil
- ✓ 1 tablespoon curry powder
- ✓ 1 teaspoon turmeric

Instructions:

1. Toss cauliflower in olive oil, curry powder, and turmeric.
2. Place in the slow cooker and cook on low for 2.5 hours.
3. Garnish with fresh cilantro before serving.

Nutritional Information: 120 calories, 12g carbs, 3g protein, 8g fat, 5g fiber.

Sesame Ginger Green Beans

Cooking Time: 2 hours on low

Serving: 4

Ingredients:

- ✓ 1 lb green beans, trimmed
- ✓ 2 tablespoons gluten-free soy sauce
- ✓ 1 tablespoon sesame oil
- ✓ 1 tablespoon rice vinegar

Instructions:

1. Toss green beans in soy sauce, sesame oil, and rice vinegar.
2. Place in the slow cooker and cook on low for 2 hours.
3. Sprinkle with sesame seeds before serving.

Nutritional Information: 80 calories, 10g carbs, 2g protein, 4g fat, 3g fiber.

Buffalo Cauliflower Bites

Cooking Time: 2.5 hours on low

Serving: 4

Ingredients:

- ✓ 1 head cauliflower, cut into florets
- ✓ 1/2 cup buffalo sauce (gluten-free)
- ✓ 1/4 cup melted dairy-free butter
- ✓ 1 teaspoon garlic powder

Instructions:

1. Toss cauliflower in buffalo sauce, melted butter, and garlic powder.
2. Place in the slow cooker and cook on low for 2.5 hours.
3. Serve with dairy-free ranch for dipping.

Nutritional Information: 120 calories, 10g carbs, 2g protein, 8g fat, 4g fiber.

Ratatouille

Cooking Time: 3 hours on low

Serving: 6

Ingredients:

- ✓ 1 eggplant, diced
- ✓ 2 zucchinis, sliced
- ✓ 1 bell pepper, diced
- ✓ 1 onion, chopped
- ✓ 2 cups tomato sauce

Instructions:

1. Layer eggplant, zucchinis, bell pepper, onion, and tomato sauce in the slow cooker.
2. Cook on low for 3 hours.
3. Garnish with fresh basil before serving.

Nutritional Information: 120 calories, 25g carbs, 3g protein, 1g fat, 7g fiber.

CHAPTER 8

28 DAY MEAL PLAN

Day 1:

- ✓ Breakfast: Quinoa Porridge with Berries
- ✓ Lunch: Slow Cooker Lentil Soup
- ✓ Dinner: Herb-Crusted Lamb Roast with Rosemary Parmesan Polenta
- ✓ Snack: Cinnamon Maple Glazed Carrots

Day 2:

- ✓ Breakfast: Gluten-Free Banana Pancakes
- ✓ Lunch: Quinoa and Black Bean Stuffed Peppers
- ✓ Dinner: Lemon Garlic Chicken with Artichokes and Garlic Herb Mashed Potatoes
- ✓ Snack: Buffalo Cauliflower Bites

Day 3:

- ✓ Breakfast: Greek Yogurt Parfait with Granola
- ✓ Lunch: Vegetarian Tikka Masala with Cauliflower Rice
- ✓ Dinner: Shrimp Scampi Risotto
- ✓ Snack: Sesame Ginger Green Beans

Day 4:

- ✓ Breakfast: Spinach and Feta Omelets
- ✓ Lunch: Sweet Potato and Chickpea Curry
- ✓ Dinner: Beef Bourguignon
- ✓ Snack: Quinoa and Vegetable Stuffed Peppers

Day 5:

- ✓ Breakfast: Chocolate Banana Smoothie
- ✓ Lunch: Mushroom and Spinach Risotto
- ✓ Dinner: Salmon with Dill Cream Sauce and Rosemary Parmesan Polenta
- ✓ Snack: Cranberry Orange Sauce with Rice Cakes

Day 6:

- ✓ Breakfast: Slow Cooker Oatmeal with Apples and Almonds
- ✓ Lunch: Butternut Squash and Coconut Soup
- ✓ Dinner: Mushroom and Spinach Stuffed Chicken with Quinoa
- ✓ Snack: Garlic Herb Mashed Potatoes

Day 7:

- ✓ Breakfast: Gluten-Free Blueberry Muffins
- ✓ Lunch: Eggplant and Tomato Casserole
- ✓ Dinner: Lobster Bisque with Cinnamon Maple Glazed Carrots
- ✓ Snack: Cucumber Slices with Hummus

Day 8:

- ✓ Breakfast: Greek Yogurt with Honey and Mixed Berries
- ✓ Lunch: Chickpea and Vegetable Tagine with Quinoa
- ✓ Dinner: Vegetarian Stuffed Bell Peppers
- ✓ Snack: Rosemary Parmesan Polenta

Day 9:

- ✓ Breakfast: Gluten-Free Banana Pancakes
- ✓ Lunch: Mexican Quinoa Casserole
- ✓ Dinner: Coq au Vin with Garlic Herb Mashed Potatoes
- ✓ Snack: Curry Roasted Cauliflower

Day 10:

- ✓ Breakfast: Quinoa Porridge with Berries
- ✓ Lunch: Ratatouille
- ✓ Dinner: Vegetarian Chili with Sweet Potatoes
- ✓ Snack: Sesame Ginger Green Beans

Day 11:

- ✓ Breakfast: Chocolate Banana Smoothie
- ✓ Lunch: Chickpea and Vegetable Tagine with Quinoa
- ✓ Dinner: Chocolate Lava Cake (as a special treat)
- ✓ Snack: Quinoa and Vegetable Stuffed Peppers

Day 12:

- ✓ Breakfast: Slow Cooker Oatmeal with Apples and Almonds
- ✓ Lunch: Mushroom and Spinach Risotto
- ✓ Dinner: Herb-Crusted Lamb Roast with Rosemary Parmesan Polenta
- ✓ Snack: Cinnamon Maple Glazed Carrots

Day 13:

- ✓ Breakfast: Greek Yogurt Parfait with Granola
- ✓ Lunch: Butternut Squash and Coconut Soup
- ✓ Dinner: Lemon Garlic Chicken with Artichokes and Garlic Herb Mashed Potatoes
- ✓ Snack: Buffalo Cauliflower Bites

Day 14:

- ✓ Breakfast: Spinach and Feta Omelets
- ✓ Lunch: Quinoa and Black Bean Stuffed Peppers
- ✓ Dinner: Shrimp Scampi Risotto
- ✓ Snack: Cranberry Orange Sauce with Rice Cakes

Day 15:

- ✓ Breakfast: Gluten-Free Blueberry Muffins
- ✓ Lunch: Vegetarian Stuffed Bell Peppers
- ✓ Dinner: Mushroom and Spinach Stuffed Chicken with Quinoa
- ✓ Snack: Garlic Herb Mashed Potatoes

Day 16:

- ✓ Breakfast: Gluten-Free Banana Pancakes
- ✓ Lunch: Sweet Potato and Chickpea Curry
- ✓ Dinner: Beef Bourguignon
- ✓ Snack: Sesame Ginger Green Beans

Day 17:

- ✓ Breakfast: Quinoa Porridge with Berries
- ✓ Lunch: Vegetarian Tikka Masala with Cauliflower Rice
- ✓ Dinner: Chocolate Lava Cake (as a special treat)
- ✓ Snack: Quinoa and Vegetable Stuffed Peppers

Day 18:

- ✓ Breakfast: Chocolate Banana Smoothie
- ✓ Lunch: Eggplant and Tomato Casserole
- ✓ Dinner: Coq au Vin with Garlic Herb Mashed Potatoes
- ✓ Snack: Cinnamon Maple Glazed Carrots

Day 19:

- ✓ Breakfast: Greek Yogurt Parfait with Granola
- ✓ Lunch: Ratatouille
- ✓ Dinner: Lemon Garlic Chicken with Artichokes and Garlic Herb Mashed Potatoes
- ✓ Snack: Buffalo Cauliflower Bites

Day 20:

- ✓ Breakfast: Slow Cooker Oatmeal with Apples and Almonds
- ✓ Lunch: Mushroom and Spinach Risotto
- ✓ Dinner: Vegetarian Stuffed Bell Peppers
- ✓ Snack: Rosemary Parmesan Polenta

Day 21:

- ✓ Breakfast: Gluten-Free Blueberry Muffins
- ✓ Lunch: Butternut Squash and Coconut Soup
- ✓ Dinner: Salmon with Dill Cream Sauce and Rosemary Parmesan Polenta
- ✓ Snack: Cranberry Orange Sauce with Rice Cakes

Day 22:

- ✓ Breakfast: Spinach and Feta Omelette
- ✓ Lunch: Quinoa and Black Bean Stuffed Peppers
- ✓ Dinner: Shrimp Scampi Risotto
- ✓ Snack: Garlic Herb Mashed Potatoes

Day 23:

- ✓ Breakfast: Greek Yogurt with Honey and Mixed Berries
- ✓ Lunch: Chickpea and Vegetable Tagine with Quinoa
- ✓ Dinner: Herb-Crusted Lamb Roast with Rosemary Parmesan Polenta
- ✓ Snack: Sesame Ginger Green Beans

Day 24:

- ✓ Breakfast: Chocolate Banana Smoothie
- ✓ Lunch: Vegetarian Stuffed Bell Peppers
- ✓ Dinner: Mushroom and Spinach Stuffed Chicken with Quinoa
- ✓ Snack: Cinnamon Maple Glazed Carrots

Day 25:

- ✓ Breakfast: Slow Cooker Oatmeal with Apples and Almonds
- ✓ Lunch: Sweet Potato and Chickpea Curry
- ✓ Dinner: Beef Bourguignon
- ✓ Snack: Buffalo Cauliflower Bites

Day 26:

- ✓ Breakfast: Quinoa Porridge with Berries
- ✓ Lunch: Vegetarian Tikka Masala with Cauliflower Rice
- ✓ Dinner: Chocolate Lava Cake (as a special treat)
- ✓ Snack: Quinoa and Vegetable Stuffed Peppers

Day 27:

- ✓ Breakfast: Greek Yogurt Parfait with Granola
- ✓ Lunch: Ratatouille
- ✓ Dinner: Lemon Garlic Chicken with Artichokes and Garlic Herb Mashed Potatoes
- ✓ Snack: Rosemary Parmesan Polenta

Day 28:

- ✓ Breakfast: Gluten-Free Blueberry Muffins
- ✓ Lunch: Butternut Squash and Coconut Soup
- ✓ Dinner: Salmon with Dill Cream Sauce and Rosemary Parmesan Polenta
- ✓ Snack: Cranberry Orange Sauce with Rice Cakes

CONCLUSION

As we near the end of this gastronomic adventure, I want to extend my heartfelt gratitude for joining me on this journey. It's been more than just a cookbook; it's been a shared experience, a culinary exploration into the realms of gluten-free living. I hope these recipes have not only tantalized your taste buds but have become a source of joy and nourishment in your everyday life.

In closing, let me reiterate the transformative power of embracing a gluten-free lifestyle. It's not about restriction; it's about liberation – freeing yourself from the burdens of unhealthy eating and embracing the bounty of nature's goodness. I encourage you to reflect on the changes you've witnessed, the moments of delight as you savored each dish, and the newfound energy that accompanies wholesome eating.

But our journey doesn't end here. Your feedback is the vital ingredient that will shape future editions, ensuring that this cookbook continues to be a beacon of culinary delight for all. Your thoughts, suggestions, and personal experiences are not only welcomed but cherished. Together, we can create a community that celebrates good food, good health, and the shared joy of nourishing our bodies.

So, dear reader, as you continue your culinary exploration, I invite you to share your thoughts with me. How did these recipes impact your life? What culinary masterpieces did you create? Is there a particular dish that became your go-to comfort meal? Your feedback is not just appreciated; it's invaluable in shaping the future of gluten-free slow cooking.

Remember, this cookbook is not a static collection of recipes; it's a living, breathing entity that evolves with each reader's experience. Your voice matters, and your insights can inspire others on their gluten-free journey. Let's build a community where the joy of cooking and the celebration of good health intertwine.

As you embark on this continued adventure in your kitchen, may the aromas be rich, the flavors profound, and the moments shared with loved ones be filled with laughter and warmth. Here's to your health, happiness, and the countless delicious moments that lie ahead.

Thank you for being a part of this culinary journey. Until our palates meet again, happy cooking!

OTHER BOOKS BY THE AUTHOR

<u>MEDITERRANEAN AIR FRYER COOKBOOK FOR BEGINNERS</u>

<u>LOW SODIUM SLOW COOKER COOKBOOK</u>

<u>MEDITERRANEAN DIET COOKBOOK FOR NEWBIES 2024</u>

<u>DIABETIC RENAL DIET COOKBOOK FOR NEWLY DAIGNOSED</u>

<u>RENAL DIET AIR FRYER COOKBOOK FOR SENIORS</u>

<u>KIDNEY DISEASE DIET COOKBOOK FOR WOMEN</u>

<u>GLUTEN-FREE AIR FRYER COOKBOOK</u>

<u>GLUTEN-FREE INSTANT POT COOKBOOK</u>

10 SPECIAL OCCASION RECIPES

Herb-Crusted Lamb Roast

Cooking Time: 5 hours on low

Serving: 8

Ingredients:

- ✓ 4 lbs lamb roast
- ✓ 3 cloves garlic, minced
- ✓ 2 tablespoons fresh rosemary, chopped
- ✓ 2 tablespoons fresh thyme, chopped
- ✓ Salt and pepper to taste

Instructions:

1. Rub lamb with garlic, rosemary, thyme, salt, and pepper.
2. Place in the slow cooker and cook on low for 5 hours.
3. Rest before slicing and serving.

Nutritional Information: 320 calories, 0g carbs, 45g protein, 15g fat, 0g fiber.

Lemon Garlic Chicken with Artichokes

Cooking Time: 4 hours on low

Serving: 6

Ingredients:

- ✓ 3 lbs chicken thighs, bone-in, skin-on
- ✓ 4 cloves garlic, minced
- ✓ Juice of 2 lemons
- ✓ 1 can artichoke hearts, drained
- ✓ 1 teaspoon dried oregano

Instructions:

1. Season chicken with garlic, lemon juice, oregano, salt, and pepper.
2. Arrange in the slow cooker with artichoke hearts and cook on low for 4 hours.
3. Garnish with fresh parsley before serving.

Nutritional Information: 280 calories, 5g carbs, 30g protein, 15g fat, 2g fiber.

Shrimp Scampi Risotto

Cooking Time: 2.5 hours on low

Serving: 4

Ingredients:

- ✓ 1 cup Arborio rice
- ✓ 1 lb large shrimp, peeled and deveined
- ✓ 4 cups chicken broth
- ✓ 1/2 cup dry white wine
- ✓ 4 tablespoons butter

Instructions:

1. Combine rice, shrimp, broth, wine, and butter in the slow cooker.
2. Cook on low for 2.5 hours, stirring occasionally.
3. Finish with grated Parmesan and lemon zest before serving.

Nutritional Information: 350 calories, 40g carbs, 20g protein, 12g fat, 1g fiber.

Beef Bourguignon

Cooking Time: 6 hours on low

Serving: 6

Ingredients:

- ✓ 2.5 lbs beef stew meat
- ✓ 1 onion, chopped
- ✓ 2 carrots, sliced
- ✓ 2 cups red wine
- ✓ 3 tablespoons tomato paste

Instructions:

1. Brown beef in a skillet; transfer to the slow cooker.
2. Add onion, carrots, wine, tomato paste, salt, and pepper.
3. Cook on low for 6 hours.
4. Serve over mashed potatoes or polenta.

Nutritional Information: 380 calories, 10g carbs, 35g protein, 18g fat, 2g fiber.

Salmon with Dill Cream Sauce

Cooking Time: 2.5 hours on low

Serving: 4

Ingredients:

- ✓ 4 salmon fillets
- ✓ 1 cup chicken broth
- ✓ 1/2 cup dry white wine
- ✓ 1/4 cup chopped fresh dill
- ✓ 1/2 cup heavy cream

Instructions:

1. Place salmon in the slow cooker.
2. Mix broth, wine, and dill; pour over salmon.
3. Cook on low for 2.5 hours.
4. Stir in cream before serving.

Nutritional Information: 320 calories, 2g carbs, 30g protein, 20g fat, 0g fiber.

Mushroom and Spinach Stuffed Chicken

Cooking Time: 4 hours on low

Serving: 6

Ingredients:

- ✓ 6 boneless, skinless chicken breasts
- ✓ 2 cups baby spinach
- ✓ 1 cup mushrooms, chopped
- ✓ 1 cup feta cheese, crumbled
- ✓ 1 teaspoon dried thyme

Instructions:

1. Flatten chicken breasts and stuff with spinach, mushrooms, and feta.
2. Arrange in the slow cooker, sprinkle with thyme, and cook on low for 4 hours.
3. Serve with a side of quinoa or rice.

Nutritional Information: 280 calories, 5g carbs, 35g protein, 12g fat, 2g fiber.

Lobster Bisque

Cooking Time: 3 hours on low

Serving: 4

Ingredients:

- ✓ 2 lobster tails, shelled and chopped
- ✓ 1 onion, chopped
- ✓ 2 carrots, sliced
- ✓ 3 cups seafood or chicken broth
- ✓ 1 cup heavy cream

Instructions:

1. Combine lobster, onion, carrots, broth, and cream in the slow cooker.
2. Cook on low for 3 hours.
3. Blend until smooth before serving.

Nutritional Information: 320 calories, 10g carbs, 15g protein, 25g fat, 1g fiber.

Vegetarian Stuffed Bell Peppers

Cooking Time: 3.5 hours on low

Serving: 6

Ingredients:

- ✓ 6 bell peppers, halved and seeds removed
- ✓ 1 cup cooked quinoa
- ✓ 1 can black beans, drained and rinsed
- ✓ 1 cup corn kernels (fresh or frozen)

Instructions:

1. Fill each pepper half with a mixture of quinoa, black beans, and corn.
2. Arrange in the slow cooker and cook on low for 3.5 hours.
3. Top with avocado and cilantro before serving.

Nutritional Information: 240 calories, 40g carbs, 8g protein, 5g fat, 8g fiber.

Coq au Vin

Cooking Time: 5 hours on low

Serving: 6

Ingredients:

- ✓ 3 lbs chicken thighs, bone-in, skin-on
- ✓ 1 bottle red wine
- ✓ 1 onion, chopped
- ✓ 2 cloves garlic, minced
- ✓ 2 cups mushrooms, sliced

Instructions:

1. Brown chicken in a skillet; transfer to the slow cooker.
2. Add wine, onion, garlic, mushrooms, thyme, salt, and pepper.
3. Cook on low for 5 hours.
4. Serve over mashed potatoes or noodles.

Nutritional Information: 340 calories, 10g carbs, 30g protein, 18g fat, 2g fiber.

Chocolate Lava Cake

Cooking Time: 2 hours on low

Serving: 8

Ingredients:

- ✓ 1 cup gluten-free flour
- ✓ 1 cup sugar
- ✓ 1/2 cup cocoa powder
- ✓ 2 teaspoons baking powder
- ✓ 1/2 teaspoon salt
- ✓ 1/2 cup milk
- ✓ 1/4 cup vegetable oil
- ✓ 1 teaspoon vanilla extract
- ✓ 1 cup hot water

Instructions:

1. In a bowl, mix flour, sugar, cocoa powder, baking powder, and salt.
2. Add milk, oil, and vanilla; spread in the slow cooker.
3. In a separate bowl, combine hot water and sugar; pour over the batter.
4. Cook on low for 2 hours.
5. Serve warm with vanilla ice cream.

Nutritional Information: 350 calories, 60g carbs, 4g protein, 12g fat, 4g fiber.

MEAL PLANNER JOURNAL

WEEKLY PLANNER

MONDAY

TUESDAY

WEDNESDAY

THURSDAY

FRIDAY

SATUREDAY

SUNDAY

NOTE

WEEKLY PLANNER

MONDAY	TUESDAY

WEDNESDAY	THURSDAY

FRIDAY	SATUREDAY

SUNDAY	NOTE

WEEKLY PLANNER

MONDAY	TUESDAY

WEDNESDAY	THURSDAY

FRIDAY	SATUREDAY

SUNDAY	NOTE

WEEKLY PLANNER

MONDAY

TUESDAY

WEDNESDAY

THURSDAY

FRIDAY

SATUREDAY

SUNDAY

NOTE

WEEKLY PLANNER

MONDAY

TUESDAY

WEDNESDAY

THURSDAY

FRIDAY

SATUREDAY

SUNDAY

NOTE

WEEKLY PLANNER

MONDAY	TUESDAY

WEDNESDAY	THURSDAY

FRIDAY	SATUREDAY

SUNDAY	NOTE

WEEKLY PLANNER

MONDAY	TUESDAY

WEDNESDAY	THURSDAY

FRIDAY	SATUREDAY

SUNDAY	NOTE

WEEKLY PLANNER

MONDAY	TUESDAY

WEDNESDAY	THURSDAY

FRIDAY	SATUREDAY

SUNDAY	NOTE

WEEKLY PLANNER

MONDAY	TUESDAY

WEDNESDAY	THURSDAY

FRIDAY	SATUREDAY

SUNDAY	NOTE

WEEKLY PLANNER

MONDAY

TUESDAY

WEDNESDAY

THURSDAY

FRIDAY

SATUREDAY

SUNDAY

NOTE

www.ingramcontent.com/pod-product-compliance
Lightning Source LLC
Chambersburg PA
CBHW080937260726
48661CB00010B/3949